CONGRATULATIONS ON YOUR DECISION TO GET HEALTHY!

"21 Days" to a New Healthy You! Hearty Vegan and Vegetarian Slow-Cooker Recipes

COOKBOOK VI

A guide to a *new healthy "comfort food" slow cooker recipe plan* that is not a "DIET", created based on personal experience to help you *finally* keep up with your weight loss management, weight management and overall health goals.

"21 Days" to a New Healthy You! Hearty Vegan and Vegetarian Slow-Cooker Recipes

---

A 21 DAY SLOW-COOKER RECIPE GUIDE FOR VEGANS, VEGETARIANS, THOSE WHOM ARE TRANSITIONING TO VEGAN AND/OR VEGETARIAN or whom simply want to have "meatless and dairy-less" meal days for a better *"LIFE"*

KYLA LATRICE, MBA

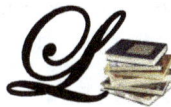

Lady Mirage Publications, Inc.

New York   Memphis   Los Angeles   London   Cape Town   Toronto
Atlanta   Singapore   Japan

Published by:
Lady Mirage Publications, Inc.
3724 Goodman Rd W, Unit 575
Horn Lake, MS 38637
www.LadyMirageAgency.com

Manufactured in the United States of America
First Edition: June 2014

Lady Mirage Publications, Inc. is an imprint and subsidiary
of Lady Mirage Global. The Lady Mirage Publications, Inc. name
and logo are trademarks of Lady Mirage Global.

Authors within the Lady Mirage Global (under Lady Mirage Agency,
Inc.), Lady Mirage Publications and Lady Mirage Literary Agency
speakers division provides a wide range of authors for speaking
engagements. To find out more information, go to
www.LadyMirageAgency.com
Cover photos provided by www.FreeDigitalPhotos.net
The publisher is not responsible for websites (or their content) that
are not owned by the publisher.

Library of Congress Cataloging-in-Publication Data:
eISBN: 978-1-31-076753-1; Print ISBN: 978-0-9975371-5-4
Tennin, Kyla Latrice.
21 Days to a New Healthy You! Hearty Vegan and Vegetarian Slow-
Cooker Recipes   Pages cm; copyrighted materials.
    1.   Health-Nutrition-Diet-Fitness. 2. Cooking. 3. Fitness.
Library of Congress Catalog Card Number: 2016907246

Print Book Edition, License Note

Also Note

In this book, Ms. Latrice begins by explaining a *fast* that she has created, tested and tried, which contributed to her weight loss, weight management and healthy eating lifestyle journey.
She has also written this book due to there being so many books, health, weight-loss and "diet" programs currently on the global market. The programs and books she has seen and reviewed are too long, too thick, have too much information and many times, are difficult for people to read. This book was written to *simplify and shorten* how to lose weight and maintain your health, for life. It is based on personal experience and is still done today. It's an effective solution.

"21 Days" to a New Healthy You! Hearty Vegan and Vegetarian Slow-Cooker Recipes

Table of Contents

*Some recipes titles here have been condensed to fit the format of this book
Full recipe titles are on the pages of the actual recipe*

HEARTY SLOW-COOKER RECIPES.......................................41

Day 1: Hearty Warm Vegetarian Gumbo...................45

Day 2: Spinach & Sweet Potato Squash Stew.......43

Day 3: Lentil, Cabbage & Potato Slow-Cooked Stew....47

Day 4: Year-Round Butternut Squash Chili.........49

Day 5: Minestrone Stew...51

Day 6: Hearty Mango Slow-Cooked Beans.........53

Day 7: Apple Wild Rice Soup...............................55

Day 8: Crock Pot Pumpkin Stew.......................57

Day 9: Black Beans and Greek Rice with Green Onion...59

Day 10: Corn, Black Bean and Pepper Chowder...61

Day 11: Sweet Potato & Spinach Slow-Cooked Soup....63

Day 12: Chipotle Black Bean Kidney Bean Stew..65

Day 13: Slow-Cooked Cauliflower Broccoli Stew........67

Day 14: Leek, Potato & Cauliflower Stew..........69

Day 15: Slow-Cooked Split Pea Stew......................71

Day 16: Slow-Cooked Fennel Stew...................73

Day 17: Southern Belle Tortilla Stew.......................75

Day 18: Southern Style Barley Stew.................77

Day 19: Slow Roasted Sweet Potato Carrot Stew.........79

Day 20: Slow Roasted Vegetarian Stew..............81

Day 21: Hearty Beet Stew..83

INDEX...85

Hearty Slow-Cooker Recipes................85

DEDICATION

This cookbook is dedicated to men and women around the world that have dealt with or are beginning to deal with food addiction, obesity and/or declining health.

I also dedicate this book to those whom have been "Mirage's" in life; overlooked, betrayed, not good enough, slandered, mistreated, misunderstood, misrepresented and even treated unfairly because of their weight or how they looked on the **outside** to others, when in fact, on the **inside** there's greater.

This new cookbook is also dedicated to men and women around the world that want to
shift from being ordinary to extraordinary and accomplishing what others said you would never be able to do again or never be able to do at all.

Here's to the New You!

ACKNOWLEDGMENTS

I want to **say thank you** to anyone whom has ever betrayed,
rejected, mistreated, teased, and misused
or looked down upon me. You helped me become GREATER
and launched me into my destiny.

Whenever someone throws bricks at you, use them to *"build"*.
Build something greater; even your mansion.

And whenever you face opposition, "know" that it is actually
an opportunity; a set-back for a set-up to secure the victory,
rejection for rewards, pain for gain, lack for prosperity to
leave a legacy, misery for miracles and put downs for
promotion.

IT'S YOUR TIME...*to bounce back!*

Let's Get Healthy!

AUTHOR'S NOTE

21 Days to a New Healthy You! Hearty Vegan and Vegetarian
Slow-Cooker Recipes
Copyright © 2014
Ms. Kyla Latrice, Inc.
All Rights Reserved.

AFFIDAVIT

ALL RIGHTS RESERVED

"ON-THE-GO"

This cookbook *(and all of my cookbooks,*
books, workbook and manuals) can be read and applied in
airports, on trains, at work on your lunch break,
in grocery stores while shopping for and planning your
weekly meals, at bookstore cafes,
at restaurants *(for quick decision making; to remember your*
health and/or weight loss goals) and even in shopping malls.

In addition, *this book can be brought to*
fast food restaurants (to pull up and look through to remember
your goals before ordering), at the park (before a jog or
potluck), during your hotel stays,
on vacations and at airport food counters when ordering your
meals and drinks *(so you remember your goals and what to*
eat and drink).

This cookbook has been made available
on mobile devices via Adobe Digital Editions and DRM
(Digital Rights Management).

WORLD STATISTICS

Obesity and Childhood Obesity
Centers for Disease Control and Prevention
http://www.cdc.gov/obesity/data/adult.html
http://www.cdc.gov/nchs/fastats/obesity-overweight.htm

Harvard School of Public Health
http://www.hsph.harvard.edu/obesity-prevention-source/obesity-trends/

World Health Organization
http://www.who.int/topics/obesity/en/

Stroke Awareness and Prevention
http://www.cdc.gov/stroke/facts.htm

Diabetes Awareness and Prevention
Centers for Disease Control and Prevention
http://www.cdc.gov/diabetes/data/statistics/2014statisticsreport.html

American Diabetes Association
http://www.diabetes.org/diabetes-basics/statistics/

"FASTING"

WHAT IS FASTING?

➤ Fasting is abstaining from PLEASURABLE foods for a certain amount of time to FOCUS on things that are more important than pleasurable foods to get to the root of what is causing your poor health, obesity, relationships and quality of life.

➤ It is not a hunger strike.

➤ You're able to see into your life better and rid it of the bad when you pull away from portion after portion at the dinner table, lunch buffet after buffet with friends and co-workers, nightly binge eating and drinking (whether alcohol, sodas, sugary drinks and the like) and dessert or movie nights on the sofa with a large pizza box and donuts.

➤ Fasting helps you pinpoint where you overdo things (overindulge), gets you back on track and teaches you how to eat, "in moderation" (balance), for your health and for a better life.

➤ Your body may not like eating healthy for the first few days (especially if you have never fasted before), but it will adjust.

REASONS FOR FASTING:

➤ It produces a physical discipline (especially for how, when, where and *what* you eat).

➤ It rids the body of toxins (just like exercise does when you sweat); cleansing your body and digestive tracts, improving your health and weight.

Note: If you are on medication, consult your physician before any *fast*.

BENEFITS OF FASTING:
➢ It strengthens *you* and your body.

➢ Fasting brings joy, happiness and *energy* to your life; and fruits, vegetables, oils, etc. are quite inexpensive. Make a list and shop for your ingredients before you begin.

➢ You become very aware of *what* and *how much* you eat. You also begin to pay more attention to when and where you always eat/drink and what leads you to OVEREATING.

➢ Fasting brings humility, revelation and an overall healthy lifestyle (mind, emotions, intellect, etc.).

TYPICAL TYPES OF FASTS:
Sometimes people fast the following from their lives:
➢ Television (even the internet, social media or video games) for one day, three days or even one week, television during certain hours of the day (to break a cycle of watching certain shows they may be addicted to (like food) that aren't good for them.
           ....or
➢ To break a cycle of "certain foods" they may eat while watching certain television shows.

➢ Fasting to abstain from all pleasurable foods and red meats, eating only fruits, vegetables, clear soups, cereals (no white sugar), water, diluted fruit juices (100% juices only) and/or grains.

➢ Some people even fast people (bad acquaintances, friendships or relationships), leading eventually to moving away from those person's completely, for a better life and health. Your health is your life.

➢ Many people fast for 24 hours, three days, seven days, 14 days, 21 days or longer. My success and learning my body as well as other persons bodies (whom have fasted when I have fasted) has come from "closely monitoring" how the body reacts to each of these fasts (particularly "21 days") and I've noticed some things and have sculpted recipes to help others find that tremendous success in many areas of their lives as well.

➢ Fasts should always be broken slowly, especially if you have been on an "extended fast" (a fast for more than 30 days, a salad only fast, a smoothie only fast or even a clear soup only fast).

➢ Gradually get back into "regular food", until you can completely commit to "healthy food" (and a regular healthy lifestyle); such as having juices for a couple of days, then fruits, vegetables, grains and adding meats back into your diet last, if applicable.

➢ Typically, people have six meals per day (three main meals (breakfast, lunch and dinner) and three snacks). For each of my Fasts or Recipes, you determine how many meals. Don't worry, fruits and vegetables do not cause obesity, they prevent it. Yet, always watch your portion sizes, in general, and with soups, stews and anything that has meat included. Never eat meat in excess.

➢ You can even choose to eat one meal per day for 21 days (there are enough recipes listed in this book), a snack, have 5-8 bottles of water and be sure to get a nap in and some exercise during the week. As you advance you can mix your salad fast with a smoothie fast and detox fast by doing one of the fasts, each per week, for 21 days, etc.

HEARTY VEGAN AND VEGETARIAN SLOW-COOKER RECIPES

THE *"SALAD FAST"*
BIRTH

Kyla Latrice is a native of Marks, MS and enjoys food and traveling. Being from a small town and a country gal, she set her goals high. Graduating from a private institution with a Bachelor of Arts Degree (BA) *(women's studies and health background; pre-medicine)* and a Master's Degree (MBA) in Business Administration with **Executive Education at Harvard and Stanford** along with several certifications and nearly 50-80 self-study coursework in legal, intellectual property and self-help, she has become one of the leading entrepreneurs of her time.

Currently Ms. Latrice is finishing up her Doctoral Honorary Degree *(Doctor of Management in Organizational Leadership)* and continues to serve on Board of Directors throughout the world for various causes; still relating to her life's purpose and corporations work. Ms. Latrice travels extensively for speaking engagements in the areas of health, wellness, obesity, poverty, domestic violence, branding, image, leadership, mentoring, business, entrepreneurship and the like.

To date, Ms. Latrice has mentored with over 20 plus organizations *(from elementary to senior citizen)*, helping others overcome issues she has faced.

With her first *corporate* job opportunity being at a "Health Food Restaurant" *(when she was age 15 or 16)* to work as a deli attendant at the deli bar, hostess *(when others were out for the day)* and bakery attendant as well as a chef in the *salad bar*.

Her main role was to attend to the deli, to prepare healthy pasta salads, healthy sandwiches, healthy shakes, healthy sundaes and *healthy smoothies*. However, Ms. Latrice was blessed with the opportunity to be called upon whenever management needed her help in the other areas as well, **to continue learning**. This gave Ms. Latrice very valuable experience and a "look" into health and business ownership, a bit deeper, which still remains with her today.

THE *"SALAD FAST"*
BIRTH

KYLA LATRICE
BEFORE
21 DAY SALAD FASTS

Ms. Latrice's *(on the left in the photo)* Corporations are inclusive of health restaurants, retail stores, property and land as well as product development organizations along with nonprofit foundations to care for the displaced, homeless.

Further, Ms. Latrice's love for food turned into obesity when her life took a turn in the early 2000's during domestic violence, sinful relationships, bad friendships, emotional binge eating and more; then again in the 2000's with another domestic violence relationship, obesity slander from family members, mental and spiritual abuse, abortion, home foreclosure, vehicle repossession and much *more*, which all have an effect on health, but she made sure her Corporations still stood; to help others.

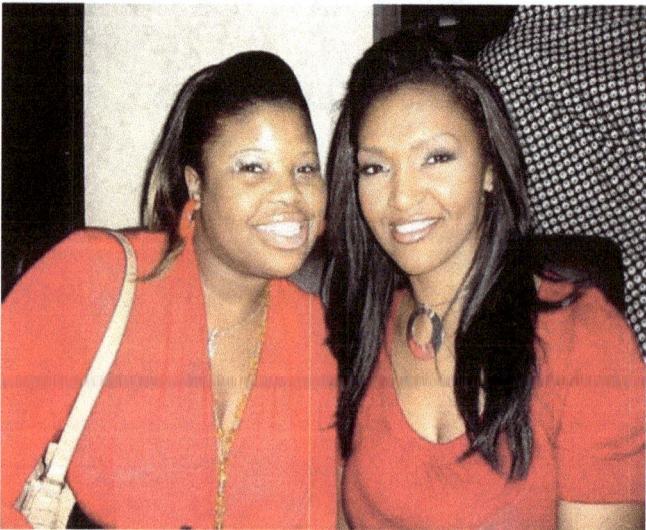

THE *"SALAD FAST"* BIRTH

KYLA LATRICE
"IN THE MIDDLE"
AFTER GAINING WEIGHT BACK FOR A SECOND TIME
21 DAY SALAD FASTS

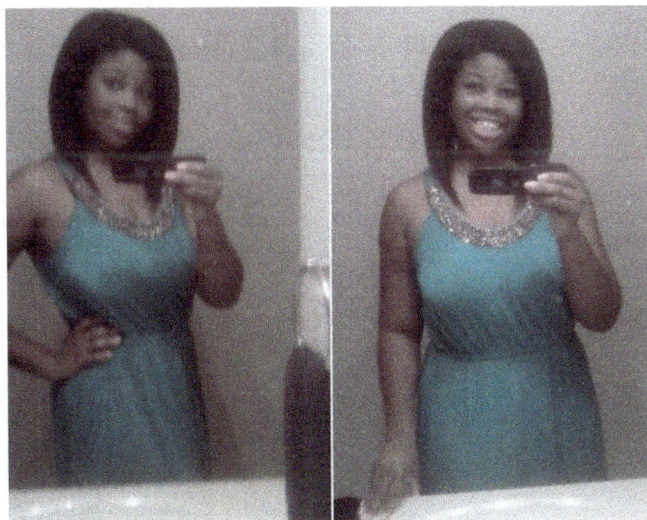

THE *"SALAD FAST"* BIRTH

KYLA LATRICE
AFTER
21 DAY SALAD FASTS

THE FINALE

HEARTY VEGAN AND VEGETARIAN SLOW-COOKER RECIPES

Many factors can contribute to obesity, such as abuse *(mental, spiritual, physical, sexual)*, poor eating habits, environment, bad friendships, sin and more. Personally, I, myself, was never taught how to eat, I did not know what to eat *(that was truly healthy for me)* and I did not know how to deal with life's problems.

Nevertheless, how can someone teach you what they don't know? My first encounter with obesity was when I was a model and went from a size 0 to a size 20/22, **weighing close to 300 pounds** *(then I lost nearly 115 pounds after prayer and seeking a remedy)*.

The second encounter was when I gained some of the first encounters weight back and went from a size 14/16 to a size 4/6 and fitting a 7/8 in jeans, losing 68 pounds. Today, I am going to share my secrets to success with you *(the birth of the "21 Day Salad Fast")* and how I made it out over the years *and* kept the weight off. Let's get started and healthy, for life!

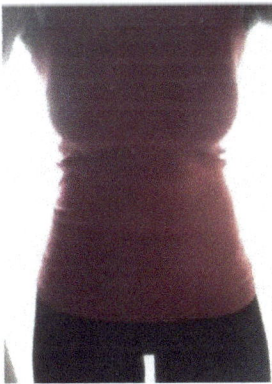

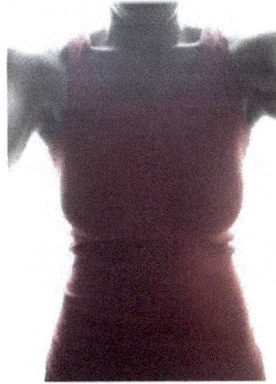

GETTING HEALTHY
LIFESTYLE CHANGE

Prepare to lose weight on the "Salad Fast" (this is not a "diet", this is an "eating plan" to reprogram your mind, body and metabolism about how to eat (portion control) and regarding what foods you should and should not be eating). It is designed to help you become healthier. Before starting this fast and any of my eating *plans ("The 21 Day Smoothie Fast" and "The 21 Day Salad Fast" as well as "All Natural Soups and Stews")*, allow yourself "one week" to prepare for the fast and eating plan by removing the following from your life:

➢ Negative relationships and friendships; they block you from doing well in life and succeeding, when people begin to see you doing well, they tend to not like it. Choose friendships and associations wisely. Be creative.

➢ Bad acquaintances; they will eventually want what you have and will cause betrayal to take place in your life through a "set-up" to sabotage all of your hard work. Always keep moving forward.

➢ Remove the following (slowly) from your daily meals (eating habits) because they contribute to weight gain (some quicker than others): soda, breads, pastas, candy bars and the like and eating second, third and fourth portions of your food. You only need one portion. Don't eat the rest!

➢ Replace all sodas with diet soda until you can cut soda out of your daily meal plan completely; only drink soda if absolutely necessary *(a lemon-lime beverage)* because there is nothing else to drink. For example, while traveling.

➢ Remove all "junk food" (cakes, pies, chips, all kinds of desserts and the like) from your kitchen.

➢ For breads, certain kinds make the weight gain skyrocket; be careful about pizza. Pasta should be limited just like soda, having it only if absolutely necessary, but once every 2-4 months is okay, just like donuts, to stay *balanced* and give your body a break from always eating healthy.

➢ Again, you only need one portion of food, per meal, work on this and you'll see results quicker.

➢ Increase your water intake to 5-8 bottled waters a day; bring a bottle with you everywhere you go so you'll be forced to drink it *(instead of something else)* and will program your body to like it *(whether you like it frozen, warm or cold)*.

➢ When you're out to eating with others, begin selecting items from menus that help *(not hinder)* your **new eating plan**, for example, order a "grilled chicken wrap with a side salad and small water" instead of a double cheeseburger, french fries and large soda. Never super-size, it wastes your results and time spent on improving your health.

➢ If you have not already, purchase my books: *"The 21 Day Smoothie Fast"* and *"The 21 Day Salad Fast"* to begin, to continue your weight loss and new you.

➢ And again, remember, commit to single portion eating, eating smaller portions (always have more vegetables on your plate than poultry/ meat), and increase your water intake *(remember to use the restroom)*. Let's begin.

GETTING HEALTHY
SET GOALS

Feel free to purchase my "A New Healthy You Workout Workbook" *(to go with your **new eating plan** and my "fasts" cookbooks* or a composition notebook from any retailer to make your own journal to measure the following (even if you need to do so at your primary care physician's office, a free clinic or go to a free health assessment machine in a retail store location that has one):

Record a written record of each:

- ➢ Your Cholesterol Level.
- ➢ Blood Pressure and Vision Check.
- ➢ Your actual Height Weight, Height, Bust/Chest and Hips size (write down your goals of where you want to be in the next week, three months, six months and year).
- ➢ Record your weight, chest/bust, hips and waist size every Saturday morning at 7am.
- ➢ Stroll through a department store and notate clothing (or take a camera phone photo) you plan on fitting into someday and notate your current sizes and then return in three months to see how you're fairing up towards your goals.
- ➢ Pick up my *"A New Healthy You Workout Workbook"* or list in your journal, your reasons for losing weight, changing your life and changing your eating habits.

- ➤ Your BMI (Body Mass Index) and where you are versus where you're supposed to be for your height, weight, age and gender.
- ➤ Bottles of "cold water" listed in the recipes section of this book are in reference to drinking 4-5 bottles of 16 fl oz bottles of water, which is equivalent to 8-10 glasses of water per day.
- ➤ Water is vital for living and for being healthy.
- ➤ The amount of water within the human body is typically 50-65% water and in infants, 78%.
- ➤ Water assists your body with digesting food and getting nutrients from the foods you have eaten to your blood, brain and other parts of your body, in order to function; emptying the body of waste and toxins, helps deliver oxygen to the body, helps prevent constipation and even regulates body temperature (in your cells, organs and tissues).

A (BMI) Chart is below for your convenience.

BMI	<(less than) 18.5	=	Underweight
BMI	18.5-24.9	=	Normal Weight
BMI	25-29.9	=	Overweight
BMI	>(more than) 30	=	Obese

GETTING HEALTHY
WHILE TRAVELING

If you'll be traveling by airplane, helicopter or private jet (smile):

> Research where you will be eating ahead of time (food choices, ingredients and prices).
> Bring bottled water.
> Resist vending machines and relying of fast food at your final destination.
> Bring your own snacks (trail mix, cashews, a banana, apple slices, peanuts) and
> Workout for free in your hotel room, taking the stairs instead of elevators and walking at the Mall.

If traveling by car:

> Pack your own cooler with ice for your bottled waters, fruits and raw vegetables.
> Consider bringing a bag of oranges & any other food that can be eaten warm or cold on the road.

If you'll be traveling by bus, train, or other means:

> Research where you will be eating ahead of time (food choices, ingredients and prices).
> Bring bottled water.
> Bring your own snacks (trail mix, cashews, a banana, apple slices, peanuts for the long trip) and
> Bring something to read or play, to keep your mind off of food and *fictious* hunger.
> At your destination, stand more than you sit (to keep your body moving) and since you have been sitting during traveling for your trip.

GARLIC

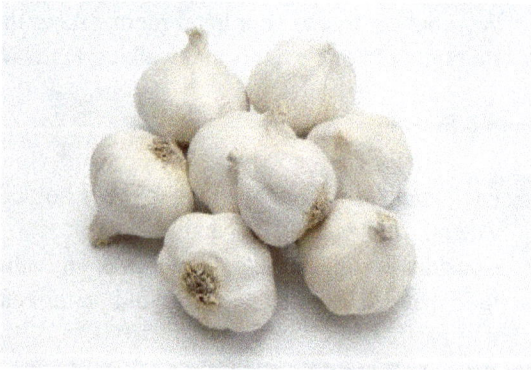

GETTING HEALTHY
YOUR NEW WORKOUT PLAN

During my both times of being obese, I never worked out at a gym nor went outside of my home to run *(weighing in at 278 pounds and trying to start my "new me" as a jogger was terrible on my knees)* to lose weight, I did it all at home, on the floor, in a compact room, near a closet. I suggest you begin a "workout regime" by doing simple workouts, such as crunches, stretching, leg lifts and a few push-ups.

Everyone cannot do cardio in the gym (paid membership prices or because of lack of transportation), running outside or bouncing around in-doors for 1-3 hours like actors and actresses on television, whom are likely being *paid monetary* compensation or by other means to film the infomercial.

Remain constant and do this 3-4 times a week, for 15-35 minutes each day. On your workout OFF days, do 100 crunches before going to bed. Consider purchasing my "Workout Workbook" to keep up with your Fitness Plan. In addition, you burn calories when you sleep, by drinking water, by exercising (which helps you live longer as well) and by **movement** (whether your arms, legs, looking out of a window, etc.).

Furthermore, water helps break down food and helps food digest. Your can also do a "mental workout" by cutting out negative people, places and things from your life.

You'll find that you have more peace in your brain and life, when you replace them with reading inspirational books, movies, community work and exercise or things you love, such as knitting, a ball game, taking a site seeing road trip (alone) every now and then or mentoring someone.

Notes

_____

_____

_____

_____

_____

_____

_____

_____

_____

_____

_____

_____

_____

_____

_____

_____

_____

_____

_____

_____

_____

_____

_____

_____

_____

_____

THE SIX MONTH RULE
GIVE IT *"TIME"*

THE SIX-MONTH RULE

On a 21-Day Salad Fast, weight [pounds] have been known to drop quickly for many people. However, the goal here is to also keep the weight off. Stay focused and be committed to at least six-months of "health work".

Remember to journal your progress.

There's something about when you write things down, they get *ACCOMPLISHED!* Also give yourself a total of six-months to work on your "New You" simply because you may lose inches first and not weight, until your weight catches up with your inches (this is what took place with me; loosing 10-12 pounds per month).

Inches first then one day the weight just fell off. And for others, sometimes weight first, then inches.

GO BACK TO THE DEPARTMENT STORE

Revisit those same department stores that you went to on the first week of your new lifestyle change, try on new clothing sizes to see where you are with your goals.

I suggest that you "mentally shop" for a new suit, a dinner dress, clothing for you next vacation (Hawaii maybe), your first pair of skinny jeans or baseball gear to wear to a game; all after you have reached your goals; to *CELEBRATE!*

Slow-Cookers, Crock-Pots and Pressure Cooker Examples &
where to purchase

AMAZON.COM

http://www.amazon.com/Crock-Pot-SCCPLC200-PK-20-Ounce-Lunch-Warmer/dp/B006H5V7ZY (Mini Crock-Pot, Warmer)

http://www.iheartthemart.com/82901/ (Triple, small crock-pots)

http://www.amazon.com/Crock-Pot-SCR200-B-Manual-Cooker-Quart/dp/B004P2LEE0 (Crock-Pot Slow Cooker, Lower Priced)

http://www.amazon.com/slow-cookers/b/ref=dp_brw_link?ie=UTF8&node=289940 (Crock-Pots, as well as Stainless Steel)

WWW.CROCK-POT.COM
www.crock-pot.com

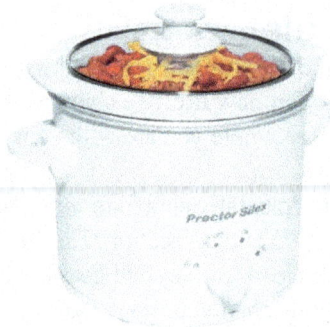

Photo Credit: Procter Silex

"SLOW-COOKER"
RECIPES

Sometimes you need to give your *body* a rest from what you have been eating regularly, *such as meats*, especially those that take quite a bit of time to digest and to rid the body of toxins that came in through certain foods eaten.

Here are some of my favorite vegan and vegetarian recipes that I have created to help you get the food rest you need, whether for a day, week or even month; to enjoy "other" foods and ways of cooking. Variety in life is good. Enjoy!

Cooking Tip:
For recipes that involve carrots, save the green leaf at the top of the carrot for making pestos
(for salads and sandwiches).

HEARTY WARM
VEGETARIAN GUMBO

DAY 1
(HEARTY WARM VEGETARIAN GUMBO)

Typically makes 4-6 servings and lasts a few days, but utilize a "Small" Slow Cooker Crock Pot or "Small Sized Pressure Cooker" (for best results) for smaller portions to watch your weight, sodium (salt) intake and to prevent over-eating

Add 1 cup of fried okra into a small slow cook crock pot or pressure cooker (select the "slow cook" button), Add 1 cup of diced onion, Add 1 cup of diced green bell pepper, Add 1 cup of diced red bell pepper, Add 1 cup of corn, Add 1 cup of diced parsley, Add 1 cup of diced roma tomatoes, Add 1 cup of diced celery, Add a dash of salt, Add 1/2 teaspoon of ground red pepper, Add a dash of pepper, Add 1 diced garlic clove, Add 1/2 teaspoon of thyme, Add 2 teaspoons of olive oil, Add 2 cups of brown rice, Add 4-5 cups of vegetable stock or Add 4-5 cups of water (to bring to a boil or to cook the ingredients evenly, if desired, to lessen sodium intake)

Cook until thoroughly heated
Garnish with finely diced snow crab (optional)
Serve immediately, after cooling (5-10 minutes)

Additional Notes: **for non-vegan and non-vegetarian:**
Add 1 cup of diced cooked lobster, 1 cup of diced cooked shrimps and 1 cup of diced cooked crab (I like snow crab) to your "pot" for hearty results and an additional 1-2 teaspoons of fresh ground red pepper

SPINACH & SWEET POTATO SQUASH STEW

DAY 2
(SPINACH & SWEET POTATO SQUASH STEW)

Typically makes 4-8 servings and lasts a few days, but utilize a "Small" Slow Cooker Crock Pot or "Small Sized Pressure Cooker" (for best results) for smaller portions to watch your weight, sodium (salt) intake and to prevent over-eating

Add 1 cup of diced onion into a small slow cook crock pot or pressure cooker (select the "slow cook" button), Add 1 cup of diced celery, Add 1 cup of apple cider vinegar, Add 2 cups of diced sweet potatoes, Add 2 cups of diced Squash (any kind), Add 2 cups of spinach, Add 1 tablespoon of olive oil, Add a dash of salt (for seasoning), Add a dash of pepper (for seasoning), Add 4-6 cups of (organic low sodium) vegetable broth

Cook until thoroughly heated until the sweet potatoes and squash are tender
Serve immediately, after cooling (5-10 minutes)

Additional Notes: <mark>**for non-vegan and non-vegetarian:**</mark>
Add 1 cup of diced cooked lobster, 1 cup of diced cooked shrimps and 1 cup of diced cooked crab (I like snow crab) to your "pot" for hearty results and an additional 1-2 teaspoons of fresh ground red pepper

LENTIL, CABBAGE & POTATO SLOW-COOKED STEW

DAY 3
(LENTIL, CABBAGE & POTATO SLOW-COOKED STEW)

Typically makes 4-8 servings and lasts a few days, but utilize a "Small" Slow Cooker Crock Pot or "Small Sized Pressure Cooker" (for best results) for smaller portions to watch your weight, sodium (salt) intake and to prevent over-eating

Add 1 cup of diced celery into a small slow cook crock pot or pressure cooker (select the "slow cook" button), Add 2 cups of diced onion, Add 1 cup of diced carrots, Add 1 cup of corn, Add 4-6 cups of slice cabbage, Add 2 cloves of diced garlic, Add several cups of washed & dried brown lentils (as desired), Add 2 cups of diced potatoes, Add 4-6 cups of vegetable stock or water, Add a dash of salt, Add a dash of ground black pepper

Cook until thoroughly heated
Serve immediately, after cooling (5-10 minutes)

Additional Notes: **for non-vegan and non-vegetarian:** Add 2 cups of diced morning star farms vegetarian sausage or non-vegetarian (stove-top cooked) sausage to your "pot" for hearty results and an additional 1-2 cups of lentil

YEAR-ROUND
BUTTERNUT SQUASH CHILI

DAY 4
(YEAR-ROUND BUTTERNUT SQUASH CHILI)

Typically makes 4-8 servings and lasts a few days, but utilize a "Small" Slow Cooker Crock Pot or "Small Sized Pressure Cooker" (for best results) for smaller portions to watch your weight, sodium (salt) intake and to prevent over-eating

Add 1 whole diced white onion into a small slow cook crock pot or pressure cooker (select the "slow cook" button), Add 1 cup of diced celery, Add 2 cups of diced apples, Add 2 cups of diced carrots, Add 2 cups of diced butternut squash, Add 1 can of black beans, Add 1 can rinsed and drained chickpeas, Add 2 diced garlic cloves, Add 1 cup of kidney beans, Add 2 teaspoons of garlic powder, Add 1 teaspoon of dried oregano, Add 2 cups of (organic low sodium) vegetable broth, Add 1 cup of chopped cilantro, Add 2 tablespoons of tomato paste, Add 1 whole lemon squeezed, Add a dash of salt, Add a dash of pepper, Add a dash of chili powder, Add a dash of cayenne pepper, Garnish at the end with shredded cheddar cheese (or grated Cracker Barrel Cheese), chopped parsley and 1 tablespoon of sour cream

Cook until thoroughly heated (for 4-8 hours in crock pot (slow cook) or done sooner in pressure cooker)
Serve immediately, after cooling (5-10 minutes)

Additional Notes: **for non-vegan and non-vegetarian:** Add 2 cups of diced morning star farms vegetarian sausage or non-vegetarian (stove-top cooked) turkey sausage to your "pot" for hearty results. Add additional (organic low sodium) vegetable broth (as desired) to thicken the chili as it cooks (keep checking) and to keep it from drying out while cooking

MINESTRONE STEW

DAY 5
(MINESTRONE STEW)

Typically makes 4-8 servings and lasts a few days, but utilize a "Small" Slow Cooker Crock Pot or "Small Sized Pressure Cooker" (for best results) for smaller portions to watch your weight, sodium (salt) intake and to prevent over-eating

Add 1 whole diced white onion into a small slow cook crock pot or pressure cooker (select the "slow cook" button), Add 2 teaspoons of olive oil, Add 2 cups of diced carrots, Add 2 cups of diced green onions, Add 1 cup of diced red peppers, Add 2 cups of chopped kale, Add 1/2 cup of chopped zucchini, Add 1/2 cup of chopped artichoke, Add 1/2 cup of chopped eggplant, Add 2 bay leaves, Add 2 diced garlic cloves, Add a dash of salt, Add a dash of fresh ground black pepper, Add 1 cup of diced roma tomatoes, Add 3 cups of rinsed and drained white beans, Cook 2 cups of whole wheat elbow (or even my favorite, "bow tie") pasta separately and then add to the crock pot 5 minutes to the end of the slow cooking (so the pasta doesn't get soggy)

Cook until thoroughly heated
Garnish with shredded or grated parmesan cheese
Serve immediately, after cooling (5-10 minutes)

Additional Notes: **for non-vegan and non-vegetarian:** Add 2 cups of [any] cut round spicy Cajun sausage or Hillshire Farms sausage to your "pot" for hearty results

HEARTY MANGO SLOW-COOKED KIDNEY BEANS

DAY 6
(HEARTY MANGO SLOW-COOKED KIDNEY BEANS)

Typically makes 4-8 servings and lasts a few days, but utilize a "Small" Slow Cooker Crock Pot or "Small Sized Pressure Cooker" (for best results) for smaller portions to watch your weight, sodium (salt) intake and to prevent over-eating

Add 2 whole cans of Kidney Beans into a small slow cook crock pot or pressure cooker (select the "slow cook" button), Add 1 whole diced white onion, Add 1 whole diced mango, Add 1 cup of Hickory Honey Barbecue Sauce, Add a dash of salt, Add a dash of fresh ground black pepper, Add 2 cups of water, Add the juice from 1 whole lemon, Add 1/4 teaspoon of chipotle powder

Cook until thoroughly heated (2-4 hours and until the sauce is thick and flows)
Garnish with a small portion of diced red bell pepper
Serve immediately, after cooling (5-10 minutes)

Additional Notes: **for non-vegan and non-vegetarian:**
Add 1 cup of cooked ground turkey and 1 cup of (organic low sodium) turkey broth to your "pot" for hearty results

APPLE WILD RICE SOUP

DAY 7
(APPLE WILD RICE SOUP)

Typically makes 4-8 servings and lasts a few days, but utilize a "Small" Slow Cooker Crock Pot or "Small Sized Pressure Cooker" (for best results) for smaller portions to watch your weight, sodium (salt) intake and to prevent over-eating

Add 2 cups of (organic low sodium) vegetable broth into a small slow cook crock pot or pressure cooker (select the "slow cook" button), Add 1-2 cups of wild rice, Add 1/2 cup of chopped parsley, Add 1 diced garlic clove, Add a dash of salt, Add a dash of fresh ground black pepper, Add 2 tablespoons of olive oil, Add 1 whole diced white onion, Add 1/2 of an apple (diced), Add 2 large diced carrot stalks, Add 2 large diced celery stalks

Cook until thoroughly heated (4-6 hours on slow; continue checking to prevent over cooking)
Serve immediately, after cooling (5-10 minutes)

Additional Notes: **for non-vegan and non-vegetarian:**
Add 2 Baked pulled chicken breasts and 1/2 cup of (organic low sodium) chicken broth to your "pot" for hearty results

CROCK POT
PUMPKIN STEW

DAY 8
(CROCK POT PUMPKIN STEW)

Typically makes 4-8 servings and lasts a few days, but utilize a "Small" Slow Cooker Crock Pot or "Small Sized Pressure Cooker" (for best results) for smaller portions to watch your weight, sodium (salt) intake and to prevent over-eating **Roast no more than 4 cups of diced (cubes) of pumpkin in the oven with olive oil and a small amount of salt for 20-30 minutes until brown and tender

Add 3-4 cups of (already roasted) pumpkin into a small slow cook crock pot or pressure cooker (select the "slow cook" button), Add 1 cup of diced white onion, Add 2-3 tablespoons of olive oil, Add a dash of salt, Add lime juice (the juice from 1 whole lime), Add 1 tablespoon of fresh [diced] thyme, Add 2-3 cups of vegetable stock, Add 1 cup of diced red bell pepper, Add 2 diced garlic cloves

Cook until thoroughly heated
Serve immediately, after cooling (5-10 minutes)

Additional Notes: **for non-vegan and non-vegetarian:** Add 2 baked pulled chicken breasts to your "pot" for hearty results

BLACK BEANS AND GREEK RICE WITH GREEN ONION

DAY 9
(BLACK BEANS AND GREEK RICE
WITH GREEN ONION)

Typically makes 4-8 servings and lasts a few days, but utilize a "Small" Slow Cooker Crock Pot or "Small Sized Pressure Cooker" (for best results) for smaller portions to watch your weight, sodium (salt) intake and to prevent over-eating

Add 2 cups of (organic low sodium) vegetable broth into a small slow cook crock pot or pressure cooker (select the "slow cook" button), Add 1 tablespoon of olive oil, Add 1 whole diced white onion, Add 3 stalks of diced green onion, Add 1 whole diced (small) roma tomato, Add 1 can of washed and drained black beans, Add 2 diced garlic cloves, Add 1 cup of chopped parsley, Add 3 cups of cooked brown rice (any kind), Add 2 tablespoons of Greek seasoning, Add 1 whole diced red bell pepper, Add the juice from 1 whole lemon (squeezed), Add a dash of dried oregano, Add a dash of salt, Add a dash of fresh ground black pepper

Cook until thoroughly heated
Serve immediately, after cooling (5-10 minutes)

Additional Notes: **for non-vegan and non-vegetarian:** Add 2 baked pulled beef and 1 cup of (organic low sodium) vegetable broth to your "pot" for hearty results

CORN, BLACK BEAN & RED PEPPER CHOWDER

DAY 10
(CORN, BLACK BEAN AND RED PEPPER CHOWDER)

Typically makes 4-8 servings and lasts a few days, but utilize a "Small" Slow Cooker Crock Pot or "Small Sized Pressure Cooker" (for best results) for smaller portions to watch your weight, sodium (salt) intake and to prevent over-eating

Add 3-5 peeled and pureed gold potatoes into a small slow cook crock pot or pressure cooker (select the "slow cook" button), Add 3-4 cups of (organic low sodium) vegetable broth, Add 1 whole bag of thawed out corn, Add 1 whole diced red bell pepper, Add 1 diced stalk of green onion (scallions), Add 1 small bag of thawed out black beans, Add 2 tablespoons of olive oil, Add 1 whole diced yellow onion, Add 1 teaspoon of smoked paprika, Add 1 teaspoon of cayenne pepper, Add a dash of salt, Add a dash of fresh ground black pepper, Add 1 cup of almond milk

Cook until thoroughly heated (Cook on low 6-7 hours and on high 3-6 hours)

Add 1 finely diced small roma tomato and 1 table spoon of sour cream to garnish
Serve immediately, after cooling (5-10 minutes)

Additional Notes: **for non-vegan and non-vegetarian:**
Add ground turkey rolled into meatballs (cooked in the oven for 20 minutes to brown) to the crock pot for hearty results

SWEET POTATO & SPINACH
SLOW-COOKED SOUP

DAY 11
(SWEET POTATO & SPINACH
SLOW-COOKED SOUP)

Typically makes 4-8 servings and lasts a few days, but utilize a "Small" Slow Cooker Crock Pot or "Small Sized Pressure Cooker" (for best results) for smaller portions to watch your weight, sodium (salt) intake and to prevent over-eating

Add 3-5 peeled and diced (into small cubes) sweet potatoes into a small slow cook crock pot or pressure cooker (select the "slow cook" button), Add 3-4 cups of (organic low sodium) vegetable broth, Add 3 diced carrots, Add 2 garlic cloves, Add 1 small bag of rinsed and dried spinach, Add a dash of salt, Add a dash of fresh ground black pepper, Add package spinach seasoning to taste

Cook until thoroughly heated (Cook on low 4-8 hours)
Serve immediately, after cooling (5-10 minutes)

Additional Notes: **for non-vegan and non-vegetarian:**
Add ground turkey rolled into meatballs (cooked in the oven for 20 minutes to brown) to the crock pot for hearty results

CHIPOTLE BLACK BEAN KIDNEY BEAN STEW

DAY 12
(CHIPOTLE BLACK BEAN KIDNEY BEAN STEW)

Typically makes 4-6 servings and lasts a few days, but utilize a "Small" Slow Cooker Crock Pot or "Small Sized Pressure Cooker" (for best results) for smaller portions to watch your weight, sodium (salt) intake and to prevent over-eating

Add 1-3 dried chipotle peppers into a small slow cook crock pot or pressure cooker (select the "slow cook" button), Add 3-4 cups of (organic low sodium) vegetable broth, Add 3 diced carrots, Add 2 garlic cloves, Add 1 diced zucchini stalk, Add 1 cup of uncooked rinsed quinoa, Add 1 small bag of rinsed and dried spinach, Add 2 cups of rinsed and dried organic black beans, Add the juice from 1 whole lime, Add 1 whole diced green bell pepper, Add 2 teaspoons of chili powder, Add 1 teaspoon of coriander, Add 2 cups of red kidney beans, Add a dash of salt, Add a dash of fresh ground black pepper, Add packaged spinach seasoning to taste

Cook until thoroughly heated (Cook on low 4-8 hours)
Serve immediately, after cooling (5-10 minutes)

Additional Notes: **for non-vegan and non-vegetarian:**
Add ground turkey rolled into meatballs (cooked in the oven for 20 minutes to brown) to the crock pot for hearty results

SLOW-COOKED CAULIFLOWER BROCCOLI STEW

DAY 13
(SLOW-COOKED CAULIFLOWER
BROCCOLI STEW)

Typically makes 4-6 servings and lasts a few days, but utilize a "Small" Slow Cooker Crock Pot or "Small Sized Pressure Cooker" (for best results) for smaller portions to watch your weight, sodium (salt) intake and to prevent over-eating

Add 2 small bags of previously frozen cauliflower (then pureed) (into small cubes) into a small slow cook crock pot or pressure cooker (select the "slow cook" button), Add 3-4 cups of (organic low sodium) vegetable broth, Add 3 diced carrots, Add 1 small bags of previously frozen broccoli, Add 2 garlic cloves, Add 1 diced carrot, Add 2-3 cups of dried lentils, Add 1 tablespoon of olive oil, Add 1/2 of a whole white onion (diced), Add a dash of salt, Add a dash of pepper, Add 1 tablespoon of chopped thyme, Add 2 bay leaves to taste

Cook until thoroughly heated (Cook on low 6-8 hours)
Serve immediately, after cooling (5-10 minutes)

Additional Notes: **for non-vegan and non-vegetarian:** Add 2 Morning Star Farms finely diced veggie burgers to the crock pot for hearty results

SLOW-COOKED LEEK, POTATO & CAULIFLOWER STEW

DAY 14
(SLOW-COOKED LEEK, POTATO &
CAULIFLOWER STEW)

Typically makes 4-8 servings and lasts a few days, but utilize a "Small" Slow Cooker Crock Pot or "Small Sized Pressure Cooker" (for best results) for smaller portions to watch your weight, sodium (salt) intake and to prevent over-eating

Add 2 small bags of previously frozen cauliflower (then puree after the cauliflower has cooked down for about 30 minutes to 1 hour and become tender) into a small slow cook crock pot or pressure cooker (select the "slow cook" button), Add 3-4 cups of (organic low sodium) vegetable broth, Add 3 diced carrots, Add 2 large diced leeks (rinsed & dried), Add 2 diced garlic cloves, Add a dash of salt, Add a dash of freshly ground black pepper, Add 2 diced gold potatoes, Add 2 cups of diced cilantro, Add 2 cups of heavy cream or almond milk, Add 1 teaspoon of paprika, Add 1 small diced roma tomato

Cook until thoroughly heated (Cook on low 3-8 hours)
Garnish with parsley and sour cream
Serve immediately, after cooling (5-10 minutes)

Additional Notes: **for non-vegan and non-vegetarian:**
Add 2 Morning Star Farms finely diced veggie burgers to the crock pot for hearty results

SLOW-COOKED SPLIT PEA STEW

DAY 15
(SLOW-COOKED SPLIT PEA STEW)

Typically makes 4-8 servings and lasts a few days, but utilize a "Small" Slow Cooker Crock Pot or "Small Sized Pressure Cooker" (for best results) for smaller portions to watch your weight, sodium (salt) intake and to prevent over-eating

Add 5 cups of dried split peas into a small slow cook crock pot or pressure cooker (select the "slow cook" button), Add 2-3 cups of water, Add 3 cups of (organic low sodium) vegetable broth, Add 2 diced carrots (into very small cubes), Add 2 tablespoons of grape-seed oil, Add a dash of salt, Add a dash of fresh ground black pepper, Add 1/2 of a diced white onion (finely diced), Add 1/2 cup of finely diced cilantro

Cook until thoroughly heated (Cook on low 6-8 hours)
Serve immediately, after cooling (5-10 minutes)

Additional Notes: **for non-vegan and non-vegetarian:**
Add 1 cup of diced ham (cut into cubes) to the crock pot for hearty results

SLOW-COOKED FENNEL STEW

DAY 16
(SLOW-COOKED FENNEL STEW)

Typically makes 4-8 servings and lasts a few days, but utilize a "Small" Slow Cooker Crock Pot or "Small Sized Pressure Cooker" (for best results) for smaller portions to watch your weight, sodium (salt) intake and to prevent over-eating

Add 1 small bag of Kale into a small slow cook crock pot or pressure cooker (select the "slow cook" button), Add 1 finely sliced fennel bulb, Add 2-3 cups of water, Add 3 cups of (organic low sodium) vegetable broth, Add 2 diced carrots (into very small cubes), Add 2 tablespoons of Balsamic Vinegar, Add a dash of salt, Add a dash of fresh ground black pepper, Add 1 cup of red kidney beans, Add 1 diced celery stalk, Add 1 teaspoon of thyme, Add 1 teaspoon of paprika

Cook until thoroughly heated (Cook on low 3-6 hours)
Garnish with a pinch of salt
Serve immediately, after cooling (5-10 minutes)

Additional Notes: **for non-vegan and non-vegetarian:**
Add 1 cup of ground turkey (with diced bits of red onion rolled into them; made into 6-8 meatballs) to the crock pot for hearty results

SOUTHERN BELLE
TORTILLA STEW

DAY 17
(SOUTHERN BELLE TORTILLA STEW)

Typically makes 4-8 servings and lasts a few days, but utilize a "Small" Slow Cooker Crock Pot or "Small Sized Pressure Cooker" (for best results) for smaller portions to watch your weight, sodium (salt) intake and to prevent over-eating

Cook until thoroughly heated (Cook on low 6-8 hours). Add a 2-3 handfuls of chopped sundried tomatoes into a small slow cook crock pot or pressure cooker (select the "slow cook" button), Add 1 diced avocado, Add 1 whole diced white onion (yellow or purple will do if you do not have white), Add 1 teaspoon of cumin or coriander, Add 1 tablespoon of olive oil, Add a dash of salt, Add a dash of pepper, Add 1 dried smoked chili pepper, Add 1 ounce of feta cheese, Add 1/2 cup of diced cilantro, Add the juice of 1 lime, Add 1 can of washed and drained black beans, Add 2-3 cups of vegetable stock, Add 2 whole diced jalapeno peppers, Add 2 diced garlic cloves, Add 1/2 of a lemon's juice

Cook until thoroughly heated (Cook on low 3-6 hours)
Garnish with chopped tortilla chips
Serve immediately, after cooling (5-10 minutes)

Additional Notes: **for non-vegan and non-vegetarian:**
Add 1 cup of ground turkey (with diced bits of parsley rolled into them; made into 12 small meatballs) to the crock pot for hearty results

SOUTHERN STYLE
BARLEY STEW

DAY 18
(SOUTHERN STYLE BARLEY STEW)

Typically makes 4-8 servings and lasts a few days, but utilize a "Small" Slow Cooker Crock Pot or "Small Sized Pressure Cooker" (for best results) for smaller portions to watch your weight, sodium (salt) intake and to prevent over-eating

Add 2-3 cups of vegetable stock into a small slow cook crock pot or pressure cooker (select the "slow cook" button), Add 1 whole diced white onion (yellow or purple will do if you do not have white), Add 2 diced garlic cloves, Add 2-3 whole diced carrots, Add 1 small bag of (previously frozen) okra, Add 2-3 diced celery stalks, Add 1-2 tablespoons of extra-virgin olive oil, Add a dash of salt to taste, Add a dash of fresh ground black pepper, Add 2 cups of rinsed barley and 1-2 tablespoons of chopped fresh thyme

Cook until thoroughly heated (Cook on low 6-8 hours)
Garnish with fresh diced parsley
Serve immediately, after cooling (5-10 minutes)

Additional Notes: **for non-vegan and non-vegetarian:**
Add 1 cup of ground beef (previously cooked on a stove top, until browned, for a "Beef Barley" type of stew) to the crock pot for hearty results

SLOW ROASTED SWEET POTATO CARROT STEW

DAY 19
(SLOW ROASTED SWEET POTATO CARROT STEW)

Typically makes 4-6 servings and lasts a few days, but utilize a "Small" Slow Cooker Crock Pot or "Small Sized Pressure Cooker" (for best results) for smaller portions to watch your weight, sodium (salt) intake and to prevent over-eating

Add 4 (previously peeled) diced sweet potatoes, 1 tablespoon of grape-seed oil, 1 whole diced white onion, 2-3 cups of (organic low sodium) vegetable stock broth, 1/2 teaspoon of curry powder, 1 tablespoon of grated ginger, 1/2 cup of diced cilantro, Add 1 whole diced carrot, 1-2 cups of coconut milk, 2-3 diced garlic cloves and 1/2 of a finely diced red bell pepper **into a blender to blend, then pour the mixture into a small slow cook crock pot** or pressure cooker (select the "slow cook" button), Add a dash of salt to taste, Add a dash of fresh ground black pepper

Cook until thoroughly heated (Cook on low 3-6 hours)
Garnish with cilantro and sunflower seeds
Serve immediately, after cooling (5-10 minutes)

Additional Notes: **for non-vegan and non-vegetarian:**
Add 1 cup of shrimp (previously cooked on a stove top, until tender, chopped, for a "Shrimp Infused Stew") to the crock pot for hearty results

SLOW ROASTED
VEGETARIAN STEW

DAY 20
(SLOW ROASTED VEGETARIAN STEW)

Typically makes 4-8 servings and lasts a few days, but utilize a "Small" Slow Cooker Crock Pot or "Small Sized Pressure Cooker" (for best results) for smaller portions to watch your weight, sodium (salt) intake and to prevent over-eating

Add a large can of crushed tomatoes (or chop them yourself) into a small slow cook crock pot or pressure cooker (select the "slow cook" button), Add 1 whole diced white onion (yellow or purple will do if you do not have white), Add 2-3 cups of vegetable stock, Add 1 cup of diced zucchini, Add 1 cup of (previously frozen) washed and rinsed pinto beans, Add 1/2 bag of (previously frozen) broccoli, Add 1 diced carrot, Add 1/2 of a diced beat, Add 1/2 of a diced yellow bell pepper, Add 1 small bag of (previously frozen) white beans, Add 1 small cup of mushrooms, Add 1 diced garlic clove, Add a dash of salt to taste, Add a dash of pepper

Cook until thoroughly heated (Cook on low 4-6 hours)
Garnish with chopped cashews
Serve immediately, after cooling (5-10 minutes)

Additional Notes: **for non-vegan and non-vegetarian:** Add 1 cup of snow crab (previously cooked on a stove top, until tender, chopped, for a "Crab Infused Stew"; my favorite) and 6-8 *jumbo shrimp* to the crock pot for hearty results

HEARTY BEET STEW

DAY 21
(HEARTY BEET STEW)

Typically makes 4-8 servings and lasts a few days, but utilize a "Small" Slow Cooker Crock Pot or "Small Sized Pressure Cooker" (for best results) for smaller portions to watch your weight, sodium (salt) intake and to prevent over-eating

Add 1 whole diced white onion (yellow will do if you do not have white), Add 1-2 diced garlic cloves, Add a dash of salt to taste, Add a dash of fresh ground black pepper, Add 1 teaspoon of paprika, Add 2-3 cups of (organic low sodium) vegetable stock/broth, Add 1 tablespoon of almond milk, and 2-3 (previously cleaned) diced beets into a food processor or blender to blend until smooth. Pour all of these ingredients into a small slow cook crock pot or pressure cooker (select the "slow cook" button) and add the juice and zest from one lemon

Cook until thoroughly heated (Cook on low 6-8 hours)
Garnish with sesame seeds
Serve immediately, after cooling (5-10 minutes)

Additional Notes: **for non-vegan and non-vegetarian:**
Add 8-12 jumbo shrimp to the crock pot for hearty results. And prepare a "side" of cooked Brussels sprouts in a small dish, drizzled with extra virgin olive oil to accommodate

CONGRATULATIONS ON YOUR NEW YOU!

Feel free to continue to use these slow-cooker for lunch, dinner, during holidays or even on company retreats and for family vacations for staying fit and healthy, on a dime, without compromising your weight management and health goals with unhealthy snacks.

*Keep up the great work by continuing
on with my two newest books, "The 21 Day Smoothie Fast"
and the "21 Day Salad Fast"*

INDEX OF RECIPES

DAY 1	45		DAY 12	65
DAY 2	43		DAY 13	67
DAY 3	47		DAY 14	69
DAY 4	49		DAY 15	71
DAY 5	51		DAY 16	73
DAY 6	53		DAY 17	75
DAY 7	55		DAY 18	77
DAY 8	57		DAY 19	79
DAY 9	59		DAY 20	81
DAY 10	61		DAY 21	83
DAY 11	63			

www.ingramcontent.com/pod-product-compliance
Lightning Source LLC
Chambersburg PA
CBHW060643150426
42811CB00079B/2298/J